Transformational
DENTISTRY

Transformational
DENTISTRY

Discover the Life-Changing Power of a *Smile*

BRADLEY M. BISHOP

BMSc, DDS, MS, FRCD(C)

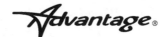

Published by Advantage, Charleston, South Carolina.
Member of Advantage Media Group.

ADVANTAGE is a registered trademark, and the Advantage colophon is a trademark of Advantage Media Group, Inc.

Printed in the United States of America.

10 9 8 7 6 5 4 3 2 1

ISBN: 978-1-59932-947-5
LCCN: 2019933366

Cover and layout design by Wesley Strickland.

This publication is designed to provide accurate and authoritative information in regard to the subject matter covered. It is sold with the understanding that the publisher is not engaged in rendering legal, accounting, or other professional services. If legal advice or other expert assistance is required, the services of a competent professional person should be sought.

Advantage Media Group is proud to be a part of the Tree Neutral® program. Tree Neutral offsets the number of trees consumed in the production and printing of this book by taking proactive steps such as planting trees in direct proportion to the number of trees used to print books. To learn more about Tree Neutral, please visit **www.treeneutral.com**.

Advantage Media Group is a publisher of business, self-improvement, and professional development books and online learning. We help entrepreneurs, business leaders, and professionals share their Stories, Passion, and Knowledge to help others Learn & Grow. Do you have a manuscript or book idea that you would like us to consider for publishing? Please visit **advantagefamily.com** or call **1.866.775.1696**.

To Tilane and our children.

TABLE OF CONTENTS

I hope you find this book a valuable asset on your journey toward wholeness. Once you have finished, please pass it to a friend or loved one so that their path might also be enriched by the journey of others.

DR. DARWIN SONG

DDS, MSc, FRCD(C), Dip. Perio
CERTIFIED SPECIALIST IN PERIODONTICS

HAPPINESS, CONFIDENCE AND SELF-ESTEEM are not the typical words that come to mind when one thinks about the benefits of their relationship with their dentist. Dr. Bradley Bishop is changing the way people think about dentistry and how their dental health can impact their lives. In this book *Transformational Dentistry* we see the positive impact that his work has on the psychological, emotional and social well being of his patients. Sometimes these positive changes come in joyous expressions of gratitude with vivid changes in the patient's confidence and behavior, such as the time one of my patient's, after having restored his smile with beautiful new anterior crowns, gained the confidence to seek out and marry the love of his life after being separated for over 20 years. Other times the positive changes are less perceptible and can be reflected in a newfound willingness to show a modest smile or perhaps an increased attention to one's appearance, such as a new hairstyle or outfit that intimates a spark of new found confidence.

As a periodontist who specializes in the prevention, diagnosis, and treatment of periodontal disease as well as the placement of dental implants I have been privileged to work with many talented dentists to help their patients achieve optimum oral health. Dr. Bradley Bishop is amongst the most talented dentists I have worked with and I am honored to work alongside him to help his patients achieve a newfound comfort, confidence and happiness.

Within the pages of this book the stories that are told demonstrate the life-changing possibilities that dentistry can have for our patients. And we are fortunate to have Dr. Bradley Bishop and his patients share their experiences with all of us.

WHAT IS TRANSFORMATIONAL DENTISTRY?

FREQUENTLY, WHEN I meet new people the topic of work comes up. They ask, "What kind of work do you do?" The reply "I'm a prosthodontist" is so inadequate because it doesn't begin to explain what I really do for a living and nobody has even heard of a prosthodontist. I have tried explaining it many ways. Prosthetic Dentistry. Crowns, bridges, dentures, and implants. Complex dentistry that most general dentists don't want to tackle. Esthetic and reconstructive dentistry. Although these statements are all accurate, they do not adequately express the true significance of the work that I do.

Dentistry is both art and science. The tools and principles of crowns, bridges, dentures, and implants constitute the important science of dentistry, but it is the art that enriches and enlivens the soul of those touched by dentistry. Dentistry is my paintbrush. My patients are my canvas. My purpose is to touch the heartstrings of each individual and inspire them to live a fuller life. Through dentistry, we inspire hope, health, and happiness. This is the core of transformational dentistry: the union of sound scientific principles with the emotional connection only possible between two people striving to create a bigger, more meaningful life.

For the last decade, I have had the opportunity to observe thousands of patients as they insist on retaining the status quo or worse, and others who choose the path of transformational dentistry. For many people, the psychological impact of a dissatisfying smile or missing teeth are sinister and subterranean. They don't realize the subtle adjustments they make in their life to feel comfortable in social settings. Or they don't realize the adaptations they make in their diet just to get enough nutrition. Some people ultimately become aware that when they look in the mirror they feel shame because of their smile, or they realize their social decisions are affected by their difficulty in eating. These are people who can experience the true transformative power of dentistry. The transformation is just as much a mental and emotional as it is a physical restoration of one's teeth.

Let me illustrate with a quick story. I recently met a sixty-year-old woman in my practice. Despite brushing and flossing and regular dental care, her teeth were deteriorating at a rapid rate. She said to me, "I just feel so alone. I don't know anybody who has problems like this, and I'm sure you haven't seen anybody who has a mouth as bad as mine." Her comments illustrate the sinister effects that her failing teeth have had on her mind for decades. I assured her that I have seen mouths in far worse condition, and that she's not alone; that, in fact, I'm writing a book to describe the process we have used to help many people in a similar situation.

This book details the process and some of the solutions that are available for people facing a dissatisfying smile or failing teeth. It allows you, the reader, to walk through the dental processes from hopelessness to success. Offering you a vision of the process helps you to be a more active participant, which in turn increases your chance of success. You can't make it through Transformational Dentistry as a casual observer. You're all in. If addressed intelligently, the challenges of aesthetics and tooth loss can be solved predictably, over and over, whether the situation is the most dire or simple. There are always solutions. This can give many patients, like you, comfort and assurance about your endeavors.

I hope to connect with those of you who are looking for a transformation and guide you through the process to make certain you get the smile you want and deserve. This book will highlight the emotional journey of dentistry rather than the technical process, and remind you that you are not alone, that other people have been in your situation. You will gain hope from the stories shared within these pages that you, too, can find solutions. The purpose of the book is to give you the confidence you need to get the teeth you want. I hope this book can be a tool to help you recognize an intelligent approach to dental problems, so that you can evaluate how your plan is developing and whether or not you're setting yourself up for success. If nothing else, I hope to inspire you to choose a skilled and knowledgeable practitioner with a good strategy, to avoid wasting your energy and your money, and sparing you the emotional pain that comes with a disappointing outcome. There is a clear path to getting the smile of your dreams, and that path consistently leads to a whole smile and a whole person. It's time to take the first step.

Let's revisit the opening question. What is transformational dentistry? It is the process by which we create hope, health, and happiness through the re-creation of smiles and dental function. This is transformational dentistry.

CHAPTER 1

EVOLUTION OF TRANSFORMATIONAL DENTISTRY

"We must meet the mind of the patient before we meet the mouth of the patient."

–M. M. DeVan

AS THE OLDER BROTHER of four younger sisters, I was raised in a home with a lot of emotions. My mother encouraged us to understand and express our feelings so that we could communicate more completely with one another. Being raised this way endowed me with skills to connect with people on an emotional level. I once had a teacher who informed my mother at a parent/teacher conference that I cried too easily. My mother retorted that she did not consider that a problem, and that she would continue to encourage connection with emotions because it would make me a good father and husband one day. She probably also knew that my comfort with emotions and human interaction would also become a critical component of my professional career.

My desire to help others and my interest in the biological sciences lead me on a journey into the world of healthcare. Early in my training, in a mixed class with medical students, pharmacy students, nursing students, and dental students, I began to awaken to the psychological impact of dentistry. As my fellow students and I discussed the care of a specific patient in class, I dismissed the importance of my contribution because the patient had no apparent dental disease; but a student from another discipline off-handedly commented on the teeth's role in psychological health. This was the first time I was exposed to the idea that dentistry could impact emotional and psychological health. As I continued my training through university, this connection was overshadowed by the technical demands of the training.

Shortly after beginning my practice at Legato Dental Centre in Kelowna, British Columbia, I met a patient named Sarah who would change the way I practice dentistry. Sarah came to me because she wanted a new smile. As I examined her, it was obvious to me that her teeth were severely worn and damaged from decades of bulimia. I struggled internally with how to discuss this with her. Finally, toward the end of our consultation, I said, "You know, there are a lot of reasons people have teeth like yours. One of them is bulimia."

She was surprised that I easily gained this insight into her life. I told her that bulimia has long-term consequences to her dental health and that any dentistry we performed may be compromised over time by the disorder.

She paused for a moment, and then looked me straight in the eye and explained, "I need this as part of my recovery process. I need my smile fixed so that I can fully heal and overcome this."

I suggested that she should first overcome bulimia before proceeding with the dental care she wanted.

She paused for a moment, and then looked me straight in the eye and explained, "I need this as part of my recovery process. I need my smile fixed so that I can fully heal and overcome this." She needed dentistry on an emotional level; she was seeking so much more than a pretty smile. She required a restored smile as an important part of her emotional journey to become whole again. In that moment, I realized the transformational power of dentistry. That is when Transformational Dentistry was born.

Prior to meeting Sarah, I'd always seen dentistry as the practice of correcting and managing dental disease. It was Sarah's emotions, and her willingness to share them with me, that showed me that dentistry was more than making sure the midlines are right and the incisal edges are the appropriate length; it made me realize that the work I was doing had much more profound effects on the human spirit than I had ever considered. Sarah's case had more to do with her mind than her mouth. It blew me away. That's where my journey toward Transformational Dentistry began. It is the application of masterful dentistry to unleash emotional growth and healing in the human mind. It is critical to connect with the heart and mind of a patient before appropriate dental care can be designed and carried out. This connection, which we explore throughout the book, allows dentists and patients to participate in profound patient transformations together.

How do we elevate the common dental experience to the level of Transformational Dentistry? First, we recognize that humans are emotional. We think we are logical—we want to be logical—but we are primarily driven by emotion. We only use logic to justify and explain the decisions that we have made emotionally. Second, we must at the very least strive to understand the emotions that stir a patient's desire for a dental transformation or the emotions that prevent a person from pursuing the dental care that they know they need or want.

Because patient stories offer the truest context for their dental concerns and problems, let me share another one with you. I once had a patient named Bonnie. I sat down with Bonnie on her initial visit, and she told me that she didn't like her smile. She said she'd already spoken with her general dentist and they'd decided on six crowns. "That's what I want," she said matter-of-factly.

I replied, "I can do six crowns for you, but is it okay if we take a step back and have a broader look to make sure that's the right thing for you?"

She agreed to this, and together we looked at her teeth, her face, her jaws, and her dreams. As we talked more, she began to tell me more about her life. I learned that she works for a company that sells RVs, so she's often on the radio and television for promotional purposes. As she opened up more, she told me of the time she had filmed an advertisement and afterward the company received an email stating, "That girl in the commercial is an attractive woman, but why can't she fix the black marks on her teeth?"

That email generated painful emotions—shame, sadness, embarrassment. It was true that Bonnie's smile was not perfect: she had various dental issues that affected the esthetics of her smile. She's been on TV for years like that, but after this comment, it became an emotional obstacle for her because she perceived her smile as a flaw, professionally and personally. Hearing what was really motivating her to seek out my services, I handed her a mirror and said, "How many teeth do you see in your smile?" She pointed at all the teeth she could see in her smile, and we realized together that there were more than six teeth affected by her concerns. We ultimately restored all of Bonnie's teeth because her concern was not that her six front teeth looked bad; her concern was the effect of her smile when she does presentations in public. If I had gone ahead and just addressed the six front teeth that she asked for in the first five minutes of our exam it would have been easier, but it would not have addressed her real concern. Furthermore, her smile would have still been dissatisfying to her because she would have six "pretty" teeth, and all the rest would look bad.

Before I met Sarah, I would have fixed Bonnie's six teeth and sent her on her way (and felt really good about helping her), but after Sarah, I learned to ask questions and listen to my patient—not just to what she said, but to the emotions behind her words. Once I made space for Bonnie to share herself, she did, and we were able to truly transform her negative image. Fixing six teeth is fine, but what was she really after? What was the real story and what was really motivating her? When I fully understood her emotional motivations, I could make sure to offer a solution that addressed them.

"I am a very emotional and passionate woman, and this has truly changed every aspect of my life and given me the confidence to conquer anything! I do not know how life could get much better than this. I feel beautiful, strong, happy, powerful, and invincible."

—*Bonnie*

For a medical field that has a reputation for being cold and devoid of human connection, I see a lot of emotions in my office. People generally come to see me because their smile makes them sad, or because they're fearful of what's going to happen if they lose more teeth, or because they're disappointed with past dental work. People don't usually come and see me because they're happy with their teeth, though they do come seeking happiness. If these emotions are the driving motivators that bring the patients in, then it is my job to hear them, address them, and give the patient the opportunity to transform them.

I recall Jim, who came into my office seeking dental implants. From the first minutes, he had his guard up and made it clear that he was not interested in purchasing any services. I spoke with him and asked why he'd decided to visit me that day. As he spoke, I listened for the emotions behind his words. When they became apparent, I validated those emotions and took them into consideration when designing his treatment plan. As we spoke, I could sense the man's guard coming down. He was more open, jovial, relaxed. Before he left he asked, "When do we get started and how much does it cost?" I was pleased, not only with his decision to follow the plan, but because we had connected, and he experienced an emotional shift, just by conversing. A barrier was lifted. When we take the time to emotionally engage with a person's story, their background and the feelings they are experiencing, we are better equipped to facilitate profound changes.

The easiest and most effective way to achieve this is by giving each patient appropriate time by slowing down. People don't open up and share until they know I care, and I can't create that without taking time to be interested in their needs and desires. When a patient feels that the environment is secure, they open themselves up for an emotional connection. Furthermore, allocating appropriate time allows my staff and myself to discuss all aspects of the procedures and answer questions, which can alleviate fear of the unknown, fear of pain, and fear of expenses.

People typically visit their dentists seeking improved comfort, function, or esthetics. We often hear, "I can't chew food properly," or, "I don't like my smile," or, "I'm in pain." It can be the color, a missing tooth, or a crown that they've hated for years. It is widely recognized that there is a correlation between a person's smile and their self-esteem.[1] As we know, self-esteem can have a huge impact on social and professional performance. The esthetic presentation of a person's smile is hugely impactful. When

---

1   Shaista Afroz et al., "Dental Esthetics and Its Impact on Psycho-Social Well-Being and Dental Self Confidence: A Campus Based Survey of North Indian University Students," *J Indian Prosthodont Soc.* 13, no. 4 (December 2013): 455–60, https://doi.org/10.1007/s13191-012-0247-1.

you meet a new person, the first thing you have the opportunity to evaluate is their face—the eyes, the mouth, the nose, the smile. When the eyes and teeth are harmonious, the face is not distracting; when you have atypical teeth, however, it is distracting. For this reason, I often refer to problematic smiles as being esthetic distractions, a term that will be used throughout the book. If you have a beautiful smile but you have a tooth missing, or a tooth out of place, or a tooth that is the wrong color, it attracts attention. It can affect a person during formative social and professional development years and can alter how they feel about themselves. If you cannot comfortably look in the mirror and be happy with your smile, that changes the way you interact with every single person and can impede your opportunities.

A lot of the people who have issues with their teeth have suffered since their teenage years and early adulthood. When we're helping them in their forties, fifties, and sixties, it's usually because they finally allocate time and the financial resources to discover a solution. It's not because it hasn't been a profound problem for a long time. One of the comments I hear most often is, "I wish I had done this years ago. I had no idea the impact it would have." It's my mission to get the message to you that now is the time to fix any issues you have with your teeth because your smile is connected to your confidence, your emotions, and your worldview. Since we understand the relationship between smile esthetics, self-esteem, and performance, why do people still wait decades to have their dental problems addressed? There isn't a single person who walks into my clinic with a dental problem that can't be solved, if we can break down the barriers that are holding them back. Once a patient has broken down their barriers to come see me, then it is my responsibility to meet and understand their mind before evaluating the needs of their mouth.

CHAPTER 2

ARE YOU THRIVING OR JUST SURVIVING?

"You don't know what you've got till it's gone."
—*Thomas Carl Keifer*

DO YOU EVER stop and ask yourself, am I thriving, or am I just surviving? It's an interesting question with subtle, but profound, distinctions to consider. The word thrive conjures prosperity, vigorous growth, and development; the word survival implies that we merely remain alive. I don't mean to downplay the importance of survival. We all need to survive, of course, but life is so much richer and meaningful when we are thriving.

In my practice, I observe many people who accept mere survival when it comes to the function and esthetics of their teeth. Teeth, however, are a critical component for thriving as a human being. Our digestive process begins in the mouth. Chewing our food breaks it down into smaller and smaller pieces so that it can be properly digested. This allows us to maximize the nutritional value of our food. Teeth are also critical for speaking. When you are missing a front tooth, you suddenly realize how challenging it is to form some words, because you depend on those teeth to speak. We require teeth for social interaction as well. Teeth help form a smile, a grimace, a frown, each time communicating different emotions and meanings.

Dentistry is a field that is inseparable from emotion, human expression, and human health. Many different problems can develop related to teeth. The primary consequences considered here can be broken down into two categories:

- *Esthetic Distraction* – any esthetic feature of the teeth that draws attention of either the individual or the people they interact with socially.

- *Edentulism* – the state of missing some or all of your teeth. Edentulism is either referred to as complete or partial, depending on whether you are missing all or some of your teeth.

ESTHETIC DISTRACTION

Esthetic distractions come in many forms and are unique to each individual. We've all met a person who has a distracting physical feature. The physical anomaly can distract us in conversation while we strive to establish a relationship. That same physical anomaly can also prevent a person from normal inter-action with other people because of shame or embarrassment. Reality is that the "esthetic distraction" does not reduce the value of the affected individual; as a human being you are of infinite worth and that is inherent. Nonetheless, the esthetic distraction can undermine the full realization or appreciation of the inner beauty of an affected individual. There are those rare people who rise to the top despite their difficulties. For the rest of us, resolving the esthetic distraction can help to unleash a renewed confidence, a new vigor for life.

"I am running for public office in my community. There is no way I would have ever even considered this prior to getting my new teeth." Lori shared this with me at her recent annual exam—so inspiring. She not only inspires me to carry on my work, but she will also inspire many other people to overcome their personal Goliaths. Her renewed confidence and vigor for life is a hallmark of Transformational Dentistry.

So what exactly is an esthetic distraction? Let's be clear that the sole objective of Transformational Dentistry is not to create glamorous smiles that you see on the covers of magazines. Sometimes that is your goal, but it is important to establish that in the realm of esthetics our goal is to achieve your goals and create teeth that are harmonious with your face and your smile so that they complement you and stop distracting you. Let's also be clear that having a beautiful smile is a natural complement to whole body and mind health. It is perfectly okay to desire and pursue a beautiful smile.

Here are a few esthetic distractions that we solve frequently. If yours is not described, it does not make it any less relevant. One person may be distracted by a tooth configuration that is not distracting to another. It can be a chipped, discolored, or missing tooth. It can be a full set of discolored teeth. The important piece is not the details of the esthetic distraction, but the effect of the distraction on the individual. Many people even have a hard time describing the details of what they are distracted by in their smile. As we go through the process of Transformational Dentistry together, we determine the nature of the distraction and from there can design an outcome that is pleasing to you.

"I think I look totally different when I smile, even now, years later. Interestingly, only a handful of people have ever noticed; it was that well done."

—*Sarah*

When we have done such a good job that your smile fits so well that it goes largely unnoticed we have achieved an excellent result. When teeth are not in harmony with specific geometric principles, they become a distraction. When we create new teeth that respect the natural geometry and dynamics of a smile, it is harmonious and a tremendous compliment to your innate beauty. The objective of correcting a smile is not to bring attention to it, but to create harmony with the beauty of the surrounding lips, nose, eyes, and face. This is the pinnacle of a successful smile transformation.

Solutions for esthetic distraction are widely varied and dependent on the cause and your specific desires. It can be as simple as moving teeth into proper relationships using braces. Other solutions include the same as those for replacing missing teeth. Crowns and veneers can also be used to change the shape, color, and position of teeth to restore them to their natural appearance. It can be as simple as whitening your teeth.

EDENTULISM

Edentulism is the state of missing some or all of your teeth. Edentulism has many consequences. When you lose a tooth, the bone shrinks; when you lose a lot of teeth, both your upper and lower jaws shrink, which causes your chin and nose to get closer together and your face to sink in. This can add decades to your appearance. Edentulism can affect your self-esteem and emotional state, but it also has serious effects on a person's systemic health. If you can't chew properly, you're compromising nutrition, but you also tax your gut because the digestive process is supposed to begin in the mouth. If you pass food on without the important digestive step of chewing, you're passing a great burden onto other parts of the digestive system. This can create myriad health issues.

There are certain patterns of missing teeth that are common. For instance, if you are missing your back teeth, it is difficult to eat many foods. You can't properly eat meat or raw vegetables, so you're stuck eating nutrient-poor staples such as bread and grains. You can get enough nutrition to survive, but they're not enough for you to thrive. This creates a huge nutritional compromise. When you are missing your back teeth, you also have a loss of support for the structures of the jaw joint or temporomandibular joint (TMJ). Missing your back teeth causes esthetic distractions, compromised nutrition, and instability of your jaw joint.

Edentulism is managed by three different solutions: bridges, implants, or dentures. A bridge is provided by preparing the teeth on either side of a missing tooth/teeth for a crown and then building a false tooth/teeth as a bridge between the two crowns. This provides function similar to natural teeth, but requires the preparation of teeth beside the missing tooth, that may not necessarily need a crown otherwise. A bridge also means that the tooth replacement is dependent on the health of the supporting teeth.

A dental implant is a small titanium support that is placed into the bone of the jaw. We can build a single tooth on the implant, a bridge, or attach dentures to reduce the amount of movement in the denture.

A denture can be fabricated in both a complete and partial form to replace all or some of the teeth.

This is a great alternative to missing teeth because esthetically they look awesome, but the function of a denture never comes close to natural teeth because dentures and partial dentures move. Lower dentures are particularly frustrating for people. The person who's been wearing a denture for thirty years finds themselves in a situation where, no matter how well a denture fits, it moves. As you lose all of your lower teeth, there's huge resorption of the jaw bone. There's nothing holding the denture in place, so the tongue is constantly bumping it around. Eating with a piece of plastic floating around your mouth is difficult. Dentures are the traditional solution for complete edentulism, and are better alternatives to no teeth, but they are not great substitutes for providing a high quality of life. Because dentures move, there is often a compromise in the efficiency of nutrition and, possibly, jaw joints.

A huge aspect of edentulism that is often over-looked is the emotional component—namely the feeling of being a whole person. When you are missing teeth, you may be ashamed of your smile. You may spit when you speak. You may feel like you can't go out to eat with friends anymore because you can't properly chew food.

When a person has a new set of teeth, they experience a renewed vigor because all of a sudden, they can eat things they want to, without compromising the way they're chewing. They can go out to eat, smile freely, and speak in public without worrying about their teeth moving or falling. The best solutions create teeth that don't move.

As we will discover, these two realms of dentistry—esthetic distraction and edentulism—are often related and overlapping. The major differences lie in whether the issues compromise the physical health or emotional health. Who is to say which one is a more profound compromise?

There are many reasons why people might have edentulism or esthetic distraction, so let's consider the most common causes.

CAUSES OF EDENTULISM AND ESTHETIC DISTRACTION

- Trauma/Injury

- Tooth Decay

- Grinding Teeth

- Periodontal Disease

- Developmental Disorders

TRAUMA/INJURY

Dental trauma or injury occurs in many different ways. Frequently, athletic endeavors such as hockey, quading, biking, or even tennis can result in traumatic injury of the front teeth. Some of the worst injuries I have seen are related to motor vehicle accidents and involve severe facial trauma. Injuries can range from having a chipped front tooth to having entire teeth knocked right out of the mouth. These can be the most devastating causes of edentulism and esthetic distraction because they occur suddenly without any warning. A person's identity and function can change in an instant without any preparation.

I treated one patient who was missing his front teeth and refused to tell me why. Later, after he felt more comfortable with me, he admitted, "I was in college. I was drunk, and I fell down a flight of stairs." He was a physician, and he had a real complex about his smile because he was wearing a partial removable denture. Because of that one injury, he was self-conscious about his smile for three decades before he got implants. After his journey through Transformational Dentistry, he had a smile that looked great and teeth that didn't move anymore.

TOOTH DECAY

The most common disease that we deal with in dentistry is caries—also known as tooth decay or cavities. Decay is the result of a slow acidic erosion of the tooth caused by bacteria that live in all of our mouths; they feast on the carbohydrates we eat and then excrete acid onto our teeth. Over time, this results in cavities, or holes, in our teeth. Unfortunately, we cannot eliminate the bacteria that cause decay, but we can manage the effects by reducing the exposure of our teeth to carbohydrates (by eating fewer of them) and by cleaning our teeth (by brushing and flossing) two to three times a day and by having your teeth professionally cleaned by a dental hygienist.

Most commonly tooth decay affects us in our early years and in the later years of life, but nobody is immune. Tooth decay is treated by removing the affected part of the tooth and replacing it with a filling. This compromises the integrity of the tooth and eventually some of these teeth that have fillings become weak and break. When they break, they can often be fixed, but sometimes they cannot be fixed. The other challenge with fillings is that over time the filling and the tooth take on different colors.

GRINDING TEETH

We all clench or grind our teeth, though some of us do it more than others. Clenching and grinding of the teeth over time results in breakdown and loss of tooth structure. This can result in the teeth looking shorter over time, becoming chipped, or becoming misshapen. Some people even clench and grind so fiercely that they break teeth. As we grind our teeth away, they get shorter and our nose and chin get closer together in a similar way to tooth loss. Some people have ground away so much tooth structure that they look like they have no teeth, even though they have a full set of teeth. This makes us look older and it can even result in teeth breaking so much that they are lost. Dentists often prescribe a nightguard to prevent damage to the teeth during sleep.

PERIODONTAL DISEASE

There are many diseases that affect the teeth. One of the most common diseases that we deal with is periodontal disease. This results in loss of the bone and gums that support the teeth in the jaws. Periodontal disease is caused by certain bacteria that cause inflammation around the teeth in susceptible people.

The bone loss is usually gradual but ultimately results in tooth loosening and then tooth loss. Periodontal disease is managed—it is not overcome—so it requires commitment to many years of professional dental care to prevent tooth loss. Oftentimes, the teeth appear long and spaces begin to appear between the teeth.

DEVELOPMENTAL DISORDERS

There are several disorders that affect the development of teeth. These disorders, unfortunately, affect people at a very delicate age. Often as they enter their teen years, they begin looking for a solution so that they can just look normal—so they won't get teased about their teeth. Amelogenesis imperfecta is a genetic disorder that results in poor formation of enamel and therefore results in early and significant discoloration, wear, and even failure of the teeth. Oligodontia or hypodontia are conditions characterized by people missing several teeth, with some of the remaining teeth being poorly developed. Furthermore, when a child suffers from an intense fever or other disease, it is possible for the developing adult teeth to be damaged; this could result in defects in the structure of the teeth later in life. There are many developmental and disease-related conditions that can affect a person's teeth. Because the patient "looks different" in their developmental years, they often have concerns related to their appearance or have difficulties properly chewing throughout their life. This can, of course, create emotional issues and sensitivities for the patient to work through.

THRIVING OR SURVIVING?

Whether you survive or thrive often comes down to a series of decisions. As we review the various causes of esthetic distraction and edentulism, it is clear that, as with any part of life, we don't get to choose what cards we are dealt. We do get to choose what to do about it. We do get to choose to simply accept a loss in quality of life or to pursue and create solutions in our life. The rest of this book is for those who are looking for a solution. It describes the process of transformational dentistry and the experience that many people have had by going through the process.

"Overnight, I felt embarrassment and ashamed. I felt poor and uncared for. The difference between having nice teeth and not having them was very significant."

—*Carol*

You can survive without that tooth. You're not going to die, but you are not going to be your best self when you know your smile is compromised and distracting. Furthermore, it's devastating not to be able to chew properly. Suddenly, social dinners out and meals with in-laws become anxiety-producing events. One of the major motivators for preventing tooth loss, beyond the loss of dental functionality, is because of the emotional toll it takes on a person. There's a huge social disability that comes with tooth loss. You feel less than whole. When a person has a pleasing, functional, pain-free set of teeth, there is a vigor to them. They can eat what they want. They can speak and smile. The real problem of esthetics is not the anatomical or the physical, it is the psychosocial impact of their appearance.

Regardless of the reason someone comes to me seeking a change, I must listen to what they are saying and feeling, not what I'm seeing. Whether or not I think a person does or doesn't have a beautiful smile is irrelevant; what's most relevant is that the individual thinks there is a problem. How can I alleviate the issue and get them closer to feeling whole?

Use the questionnaire below to help you gauge how much your smile impacts your quality of life each day. If you find that your choices and behaviors are inhibited because of your smile, now is the time to take the first step toward wholeness. Let the remaining chapters of this book inform and motivate you through your own transformative process.

SMILE IMPACT
QUESTIONNAIRE

HOW DOES YOUR SMILE IMPACT YOUR DAILY LIFE?

Answer the following statements using the scores below to determine your smile's impact on your daily life.

1 - Strongly Disagree
2 - Disagree
3 - Agree
4 - Strongly Agree

- I am dissatisfied with the appearance of my teeth.

- I don't like to show my teeth when I smile.

- I am sometimes concerned with what people might think about my teeth.

- I think most people I know have nicer teeth than I do.

- I don't like to see my teeth in photographs.

- I am missing one or more teeth.

- I modify my food choices because of my teeth.

- It is difficult for me to eat certain foods.

SCORING:

8-16: Your smile is not affecting your daily decisions and quality of life.

17-21: Your smile can sometimes affect the decisions that you make, either socially or nutritionally, or both.

22-32: Your smile is dramatically affecting your daily life and the choices you make socially and nutritionally.

CHAPTER 3

THE PROCESS OF TRANSFORMATIONAL DENTISTRY

"Begin with the end in mind."
—*Stephen Covey*

WHEN ERNIE PRESENTED for an examination regarding a replacement of his upper front teeth, he told me that he had just recently received a brand-new bridge to replace his lower front teeth. As I was speaking with him about his experience, concerns, and expectations, he said, "I like the bridge, but why did the doctor put it in crooked?" The bridge was indeed crooked. In fact, it sloped dramatically downward from the left to the right. I explained that as dentists, we are only trained to be technically proficient and that the bridge was well done from a technical perspective—it fit well and replaced the missing teeth. From an artistic and transformational perspective, however, it was a missed opportunity.

In dentistry, we're literally trained to fill holes. Another word for cavity is hole. When a person is missing a tooth, they receive a bridge, partial denture, or an implant to literally fill that hole.

When we consider the psychological as well as the anatomical problems, we advance dental care even one step further.

If a person needs a root canal, we create a space, or hole, inside of the tooth and fill it. I'm the first to admit, dentists are high-caliber hole fillers! When we just look at the hole without putting it in to the context of the heart and mind and face of a person, we miss the point. As we fill one hole after another, we invariably compound problems and eventually end up with a distorted dentition. This happens over decades as one dentist after another treats patients without stepping back to view a larger perspective.

Transformational Dentistry requires facial analysis and evaluation of full arches of teeth rather than only single tooth problems, for example. When we consider the psychological as well as the anatomical problems, we advance dental care even one step further. This book is my battle cry for patients and dentists to look at the big picture before doing a crown, bridge, implant, veneer, denture, or any other procedure.

So, what is the big picture? As we discussed in Chapter 1, we must first look to the mind of the patient. Where are you coming from? What are your concerns? What are your personal goals in life? What are your goals for your smile? How do your goals for your teeth fit into your big picture? Secondly, we must determine how your teeth compare to a complete, healthy, and esthetic dentition. So what does a complete, healthy, and esthetic dentition look like? In general, humans develop their central incisors and first molars before the rest of their teeth. This development pattern sets people up for the best smile and the best function.

DEVELOPMENT OF HUMAN DENTITION

The human dentition as it develops naturally is built on the position of the upper front two teeth, the lower front two teeth, and the upper and lower first molars. As dentists evaluate the teeth, we must determine that a few key factors are met to ensure that any dentistry performed is completed with the best long-term result. As we approach the mouth, we must consider what characterizes a normal dentition.

CHARACTERISTICS OF NORMAL DENTITION

1. Central incisors are in the right place. There are many artistic and scientific factors in determining this position, but in general terms, the midline between the two front teeth should be in line with the middle of the face, and the incisal (biting) edge of the central incisors should be showing a little bit when the lip is at rest. There are huge variations depending on age, gender, lip length, lip mobility, and other factors.

2. Upper occlusal plane is built to an anatomically natural plane. This means that all the upper teeth are on the same plane as each other, without any being shorter or longer. This occlusal plane is often parallel to a line that goes through your pupils. It is also parallel with a few other anatomical planes in your head.

3. Lower incisors are in the right place. The lower midline is also in line with the middle of the face, sits slightly behind the upper front teeth, and has a little overlap with the upper teeth.

4. Vertical relationship between the upper and lower jaws is right. This vertical relationship is critical for providing proper support for the front teeth and the jaw joints and the soft tissues of the face.

5. All the back teeth meet together at the same time in harmony with the jaw joints.

When all five of these factors are in harmony, esthetics and optimal dental function are achieved. When a filling, a bridge, or an implant is considered within the context of these five factors, they can be done in such a way to ensure future optimal function and esthetics. If they are not considered, the patient's current suboptimal compromised esthetics and function are locked in even further. Dentists are not trained to view dental procedures within this framework. That's why Ernie wound up with a crooked bridge.

Sarah, who we talked about in Chapter 1, was the first patient who helped me realize that dentistry has the potential to be about so much more than a simple process of filling gaps. That was my first epiphany that what I was doing, what I was engaging in with people, was so much more powerful than just meeting the technical specifications of creating a smile. This led me to the discovery of Transformational Dentistry.

THE GOALS OF TRANSFORMATIONAL DENTISTRY

- Conquer and prevent edentulism
- Correct esthetic distractions
- Transformational impact

Transformational Dentistry is less about the procedure and more about the patient's heart and mind; it is about understanding what is going on for the patient and not just with their teeth. As psychologist Abraham Maslow once said, "I suppose it is tempting, if the only tool you have is a hammer, to treat everything as if it were a nail." This is the "law of the instrument" trap that traditional dentistry falls into. Our hammer is a high-speed hand piece, and we cut into teeth and fill them or cover them. When we step back and take the patient-centric approach, however, we are no longer just a hammer.

"One specialist was totally indifferent and said he didn't understand my issues. I was extremely disheartened. I did think for a while that I would have to give up on my wish to have a wonderful smile again. I'm so glad that I didn't give up."

—Sarah

I often tell people, "I do dentistry to get to people's hearts," because as we've discussed, it's emotionally upsetting when your mouth is not right. I regularly witness the anatomical transformation from a dilapidated dentition to a functioning one. When we correct to a functional and esthetic dentition, it unlocks the heart to greater emotional transformation. The technical aspects of dentistry are critical, of course, but Transformational Dentistry unleashes renewed confidence and satisfaction for people. The teeth are just the canvas. The teeth are the point of leverage, the fulcrum that we use to catapult that person out of despair back to hope—out of feeling abandoned or betrayed, to feeling respected and cared for.

THE ELEMENTS OF TRANSFORMATIONAL DENTISTRY

Technical dentistry is developed through years of training and experience. Transformational Dentistry requires the same mastery, but includes further elements.

THE ELEMENTS OF TRANSFORMATIONAL DENTISTRY

- Technical mastery

- Anatomy

- Artistry

- Emotional Connection

Without each element, the stage cannot be set to achieve a transformation. These basic anatomical ideals must be united with the artistic pursuit of re-creating optimal function and esthetics. Emotional connection with the patient must be achieved to unleash the full transformational power of technical mastery, artistry, and optimal anatomical recreation.

For most people, one of the deterrents of complex dental work is fear of the unknown. When a patient doesn't know what to expect, they become anxious. In an effort to mitigate this stress for you, I have created phases of Transformational Dentistry that can provide you with a roadmap for care. This can ease both the anxieties of providers and patients when the process is understood and agreed upon.

PHASES OF TRANSFORMATIONAL DENTISTRY

- Discovery Assessment

- Diagnostic record gathering

- Diagnosis and treatment plan development

- Treatment planning consultation

- Prototype Restoration

- Ultimate Restoration

- Transformation Preservation

DISCOVERY ASSESSMENT

The initial phase of Transformational Dentistry is the discovery assessment. The first time we meet is an opportunity to discover what you want to accomplish with your smile and teeth; we also determine the health and problems with your teeth. The most critical part of the interview is the following question: "If you and I were to meet again in a year, what would have to change with your smile and your teeth for you to be totally satisfied with the outcome?" That question draws out what your real concerns are. Rather than me saying, "Well, here's what's wrong with you," I foster a patient-centric approach that creates an environment of communication. It allows you to articulate your concerns and your objectives. Afterward, we get into identifying what your key barriers are to achieving that goal. I need to understand if there is fear, embarrassment, or anxiety about the process. My primary aim when I first meet you is to understand your concerns and barriers. Once I can demonstrate to you that I understand this, I will begin the analysis of the face and examination of the mouth.

As we go through the examination, my job is to keep in mind what your goals are. I already know my technical objective is to achieve a normal, human dentition that is fully functional and esthetically pleasing. After I have listened to you and allowed you to dictate the narrative, I'll give you a mirror to look into while you literally point to your concerns. This helps us both identify your worries and goals.

Once I understand your self-identified objectives and move through a discussion with you, we move into the physical examination. Here, we want to identify what's going well in your mouth and what's not going well. We classify all of the anatomy that is healthy and all of the anatomy that's unhealthy. The physical exam starts with your face and considers facial proportions, facial symmetry, and evaluation of lip dynamics. The face and the lips are the smile's frame, so it's important to identify asymmetries and imbalances early on in the process so that you are aware. Next, we look at all of the soft tissues of the head, feeling around for muscular imbalances and jaw joint function.

Notice I haven't mentioned teeth yet? As discussed, we meet the mind of the patient first because Transformational Dentistry is so much more than teeth. The approach starts with where the patient is coming from mentally—what's their psyche, what's their problem, what's their objective. Then, and only then, do we consider the teeth. We work physically from the outside of the head in toward the teeth. The discovery assessment concludes by recapping your concerns, the ideal objective, and briefly summarizing our findings, which are detailed at the treatment plan consultation.

DIAGNOSTIC RECORD GATHERING

The next phase of Transformational Dentistry is diagnostic record gathering. In order to get a greater understanding of what's going on three-dimensionally, we do photos, radiographs, and models of the mouth and face from various perspectives. The jaw joints may also be radiographed to determine their health and how they are functioning.

DIAGNOSIS AND TREATMENT PLAN DEVELOPMENT

I do this often in the absence of the patient to take time to consider all of the diagnostic information and formulate the best plan to get you to the point where you have a smile that is harmonious with your face, head, and lips, with bilateral simultaneous occlusal contact in harmony with the musculature of the face and jaws.

This step is my opportunity to integrate the discovery assessment and the diagnostic records. Once I have met the mind and the mouth of the patient, and have obtained records, then I sit down in the lab to do my analysis and draft a diagnosis and treatment plan. My objective in this phase is to make sure that there is a beautiful union between where that patient is coming from and where they want to go. I consider what is actually going on in your mouth and how that achieves an ideal dentition—from a complete set of teeth to the esthetics of the smile. That will usually culminate in the development of a single plan for that patient. As part of this phase, we prepare visual aids to help describe things to the patient.

TREATMENT PLANNING CONSULTATION

The treatment planning consultation is a time to ensure that you and I are on the same page with regards to your concern and goals. We use the diagnostic information gathered to educate you about what is going on with your teeth and smile. For some people, this is a huge emotional confirmation of the problems they've been having when they can see it physically on a computer screen. To have your concerns confirmed is validating. Again, we must welcome and honor any emotions the patient experiences and make space for them to process them. The most important part of this consultation is reaching a consensus about what our plan will be to achieve your goals. Through my discussion with the patient, I'm able to assess whether that plan is truly in sync with where you are coming from. If not, I can modify that plan to be more personalized. I make a distinction with the individual that ideal and optimal are not always the same. Ideal plans overcome edentulism and esthetic distraction; optimal plans take into consideration all of the other variables, including availability of time, funding, desire, as well as addressing other barriers, such as fears and anxieties. There's a refinement of that plan to create an optimal customized treatment plan.

> *"They showed me state of the art graphics so I could easily understand my detailed oral history and what we were dealing with by way of challenges. Eventually, we had a complete and detailed verbal and written treatment plan. There were no doubts as to what would happen."*
>
> —*Carol.*

PROTOTYPE RESTORATION

In his book, *The Seven Habits of Highly Effective People*, Stephen Covey described the second habit as "begin with the end in mind." This is the essence of the prototype restoration. As we go through the treatment planning process together, we reach an understanding of what we are trying to accomplish with your transformation. In order to ensure that we understand each other, you will wear a prototype to determine if it provides the correct esthetic result and the desired functional result. Sometimes prototypes are perfect. Sometimes prototypes require significant revision. If revision is required, we are able to discuss what isn't working and what is working. We can then make the changes required to test the prototype so we know how to design the ultimate restoration. This stage is critical—it cannot be rushed and cannot be skipped. If we rush or skip the prototype, then we are just guessing how to build the ultimate restoration.

As an example, Ernie's prototype bridge should have been evaluated carefully; he should not have been surprised by his crooked bridge. Using the prototype bridge, it could have been explained to him why the bridge would be crooked and the alternate options available to him. When we put it like that, right from the beginning, the patient decides, "Well, I know it's going to be crooked. I don't want to do those other options so we're going to put in a crooked bridge." Or he might say, "I don't want it to be crooked so let's go ahead and do those other things." I am opposed to putting in crooked bridges, unless the patient has made a fully informed decision that it is the best option. This is the power of the prototype restoration, and that's how Trans-formational

Furthermore, by the choice, the patients have power. They are not victims. That is a subtle distinction until you're the patient, and then it's huge.

Dentistry handles these more complicated situations. By interacting with our patients, and being upfront and honest, we increase their knowledge base and appropriately manage expectations.

Furthermore, by the choice, the patients have power. They are not victims. That is a subtle distinction until you're the patient, and then it's huge. You might choose the crooked bridge, but you don't just want it to happen to you, without your understanding or consent. Many times, patients feel like victims. Patients, like Ernie, often come in and say, "They just put it in and I had no say." I just think, it is your face they're changing, why do you not get input? One of the goals of writing this book is to educate you so that you can get the help you need the first time instead of requiring a second, third, or fourth treatment to get what you want. For this reason, many patients come to me having lost hope. They are looking for someone to hear them and help them get the smile that other dentists have been unable to provide them.

ULTIMATE RESTORATION

Here, the word "ultimate" has a double meaning. Ultimate refers to the restoration being the final restoration that you will wear. It is also the ultimate restoration because it is the best achievable restoration based on the work we did together with the prototype restoration. Once we are both satisfied with the prototype restoration or with the changes we are going to make based on the prototype restoration, new photographs and other records are made to communicate with the lab how we would like the ultimate restoration fabricated.

Once the lab has completed fabrication of the ultimate restoration, it is tried in your mouth and the esthetic and functional results are carefully evaluated. Together, we approve the outcome. This is often a very exciting appointment. Although the prototype is a good representation of the desired outcome the ultimate restoration feels and looks so much better in your mouth. This is a very exciting time in our office for everybody involved in your transformation. The ultimate restoration provides the esthetics and function that you have been working towards through this process.

TRANSFORMATION PRESERVATION

At this point, you have made a significant investment of time, energy, and money—it is important to ensure the longevity of the transformation. Each individual's needs are different, but there are some common themes.

PROTECTION

When restorations are made with porcelain, it is usually critical to protect them at night using a carefully designed night guard to reduce wear and tear.

MAINTENANCE

It is critical to ensure that the ultimate restoration is being properly cared for including proper cleaning. Our team of dental hygienists will work closely with you to ensure that you have the tools necessary and that you're having your teeth cleaned professionally at appropriate intervals.

REEVALUATION

The human mouth is very dynamic and somewhat hostile, so it is important to have regular evaluations of your new teeth to ensure they are working properly and to prevent issues from developing. We usually do an annual examination of your mouth and teeth.

It is my hope that in understanding the treatment phases of Transformational Dentistry, I can alleviate some of the fear and anxiety that comes with an unknown process. By demystifying the process, I anticipate that I can remove some of the psychological barriers that exist between myself and a new patient. The more I can prepare you and your families, the more relaxed and empowered you become. This aids you on your journey toward the beautiful, whole dentition you've been dreaming of.

CHAPTER 4

MOTIVATIONS AND BARRIERS TO CARE

"For me, every hour is grace. And I feel gratitude in my heart each time I can meet someone and look at his or her smile."
—Elie Wiesel

WHEN SARAH'S SMILE transformation was complete, she proclaimed that she wished she had pursued it much sooner in her life because it had liberated her and helped her to feel whole again. This is why I am writing this book—to help you make that commitment sooner than you might otherwise. You deserve to feel whole again. There are many reasons why people have delayed their dental care, and though the reasons are certainly valid, I also know the profound changes that occur inwardly when someone transforms their smile outwardly. Let's identify some of the hurdles that you may be struggling to clear before you can achieve the smile and function that you long for. If we can overcome these barriers sooner, you can enjoy the feeling of being whole for a much greater portion of your life. You will be empowered to do the many great things in life that you want to do.

There are three primary motivators that prompt people to seek dental care. The first is pain—there is nothing quite like dental pain. Life is miserable when you are experiencing dental pain. The second motivation is esthetics. We have already concluded that it is not vanity that drives people to desire a natural-looking smile. It is perfectly normal and acceptable to seek wholeness when you smile in the mirror. The third motivator is function, which is usually related to the ability to eat and digest properly without discomfort. There are many discomforts—acute and chronic pains—that can develop when your teeth are not functioning properly.

PRIMARY MOTIVATORS TO SEEK DENTAL CARE

- Pain

- Esthetics

- Function

Everybody's threshold is different. For some people, a single missing tooth is an upsetting disaster, while others have to be missing several teeth before they start noticing any compromise in esthetics and function. One person may be concerned about a small discoloration on one tooth, while another may not be bothered by several severely discolored teeth. Whatever your situation, the value of Transformational Dentistry is that we are going to take the time to understand your concerns and customize solutions to help you reach your goals.

If you've established one of the prior motivators, why would you still not seek care? What might be holding you back from doing something about it? The barriers are often rooted in emotions. As we introduced in Chapter 1, we rarely acknowledge how much emotions play in our decision-making, and that applies to seeking out change, but also in actively resisting it. I hope that by explaining the process, I can eradicate some of those negative emotional barriers so that people can liberate themselves to the transformations that are possible.

EMOTIONAL BARRIERS TO CARE

- Confidence
- Fear
- Pain
- Anxiety
- Embarrassment
- Finances
- Distrust of Dental Field

CONFIDENCE

I remember chatting with a patient named Peggy after her transformation was completed. She told me that the reason she had delayed her treatment for so many years was that she did not have the belief that she would be a good candidate for a better smile. She also didn't have the confidence that there was a solution that would work for her. When you meet with a dentist to discuss your dental problems, you make yourself vulnerable, which we all know can feel uncomfortable. To overcome this, it is critical to seek care in a supportive, caring environment where the proper time and attention will be paid to you and your concerns. I often hear patients say, "I bet you've never seen a mouth as bad as mine." After years of practice, I have already seen the dental problems you have and helped many people overcome them. I promise you will not shock your dentist, nor will he or she be "stumped" by your dental issue. I hope the stories shared in the remaining chapters give you the confidence that there is indeed a solution for you.

> *"The team instilled such a confidence in me from the first initial contact and then reinforced that at every stage of the process with their attention to detail, care, and patience. They were there for me every step of the way. Each stage of the process was therefore manageable for me. I had only to heal in between. That was my only job."*

> —*Barb*

FEAR

As we discussed in Chapter 1, fear is a primary barrier to care. Many people are ashamed of how they lost their teeth, how they wore them out, or why they have waited so long to seek treatment. Some people have an intense fear of dentistry in general. Some people are fearful of the cost, to which I would say there are so many different solutions and there are ways to accommodate different budgets. In the remaining chapters, we'll look more closely at some of the specific fears my patients have grappled with and how we overcame them to achieve optimal transformations.

> *"There were many barriers that kept me out of a dental office. I have 'white coat syndrome,' with a history of a racing heart and an actual terror of needles. I also often thought, I have five children, how can I justify spending this kind of money on myself? I overcame these barriers with the help of my husband who convinced me that it was my turn. The best part of the process was looking at my new smile for the very first time."*
>
> —*Bonnie*

PAIN

Let's be honest, there is a valid perception that dentistry is painful. The silver lining is that there are myriad ways to minimize pain. We have excellent drugs to prevent and manage pain. Most of the time, the experience is less painful than what the person anticipated. Furthermore, a few days of acute pain is better than years of chronic pain. If you're in pain, then you're motivated to do something. Those are some of the easiest people to convince, because people don't like pain. In dentistry today, we can do advanced invasive procedures with little pain. Pain is something that's readily managed for most people.

> *"It's not like you wake up in the morning and go, 'Oh goody, I get to go to the dentist.' I don't think there's anybody that really likes going to the dentist. I know the process, and I'm going to put it this way: it's uncomfortable at times, but it's not excruciatingly painful."*
>
> —Lonnie

ANXIETY

Anxiety is a big barrier to care. I really feel that the careful and strategic process of Transformational Dentistry is designed to help people manage their anxiety. The first exposure is really conversation, which is not overly intimidating for most people. It draws them in to consenting to an examination. By the time we actually get to treating somebody, they've had multiple interactions with the dentist and with the members of the dental team. Furthermore, we create a calming environment: the colors are calming; the wood trim is calming; the unhurried pace is calming. The process is designed to build confidence and to help resolve fears. When the process is designed to be serene, there's time to spend with you without pressure to be somewhere else. This allows the dentist to be composed, and in turn, you will feel relaxed. We also have medications available that are designed to calm anxiety.

> *"I was terrified of the dental chair. Just the memory of those times bring it back to me and physiologically I can feel my breathing and heart rate increase. Dental work had become so stressful for me."*
>
> *—Barb*

EMBARRASSMENT

I had one patient who had been embarrassed about her smile her entire life. Once I established a rapport with her, and she knew her emotions were valid and welcomed, she admitted that she did not pursue treatment earlier because she was self-conscious— she didn't want to share her problem with another human being. The thing she needed to hear most was that her problem was quite common and that I deal with it daily. I assured her there was nothing to be ashamed about. When she learned her embarrassment around this problem was valid, she could let go of her fear and proceed without barriers.

> *"[The hardest part about treatment was] probably coming here in the first place, saying I need help, I hated my upper teeth . . . it was emotional."*
>
> —*Penny*

FINANCES

Let's face it, because of financial constraints, many people don't pursue the solutions they want. You may be one of them; you may not. I am not going to pretend this isn't real—it is real. We all spend our money on the things that are important to us. Many patients who have experienced transformational dentistry started out with an "I can't afford this" attitude. I remember Rick telling me, "Well, I guess I'm not getting a new snowmobile this year." Rick made a decision. He chose to prioritize his teeth before a new snowmobile for a year or two. If you choose to prioritize your transformational dentistry, we will design a plan that works for you. We basically use two strategies: phasing and financing.

Most treatment plans can be phased. We just need to have an honest discussion about what is realistic financially so that we can design your treatment plan to meet your time and financial realities. When we begin your treatment plan with the end in mind we can work backward to determine how to separate the entire plan into phases that work. This may mean the treatment will take more months or years than you want, but it allows you to reach your goals.

Financing can be handled in many different ways. I've had patients who come see me a couple years after we design a plan together and tell me they have saved the money and are ready to proceed. We have designed customized payment plans for individual treatment plans. Some people want to use third-party financing—this works for a lot of people.

If you are concerned about the financial aspect of your transformational dentistry here are the steps you need to follow. First, determine the treatment plan through the transformational process described in Chapter 3. Then, together, let's design a phasing plan or a financing plan that is realistic for you.

DISTRUST OF DENTAL FIELD

I often meet patients who lack confidence in dentistry's ability to solve their problem. I recently saw a new patient in my office who was frustrated and uninspired. Two years prior, she had driven six hours to a dentist who made her a new set of teeth. She thought this would solve her problem. Unfortunately, ever since she had her new set of teeth, she was experiencing severe jaw pain. She told the doctor that she wasn't pleased with the esthetics or the function of the new teeth and the doctor repeatedly told her these kinds of problems "get worse before they get better." Needless to say, she didn't have much confidence that I, or anyone, could help her. I sat with her and did the exam and I identified exactly what was causing her jaw pain. At this point, she broke down crying because she was validated and relieved to be heard. She realized it wasn't all in her head, but that there was a legitimate physiological issue that was causing pain. This is how dentistry without sentiment can be reckless, and oftentimes do greater emotional damage than doctors realize.

"The hardest part about my dental transformation was trusting the process. I had to endure dental pain my whole life with each procedure not making things any better. I still have fear deep down but it wasn't anywhere as crippling as it was before."

—Lori

There are always ways to address and overcome the emotions that people hold regarding their smiles, though it requires both the dentist's and the patient's collaboration. The naming of the emotions is not the critical piece; it is the identification of and permission to have those feelings that allows people to overcome them. Getting to the root emotions is what facilitates their dissolution and is the starting point for Transformational Dentistry. When a person has a smile that is distracting, they know it, and it affects the way they interact with other people. I have heard patients relay stories of lost confidence, recoiling from photos, refraining from going out in public, and having lost their sense of wholeness. This is why we need to get to the best solution so they don't have to suffer. That's where the transformational power of dentistry comes from, and by recognizing it and focusing on it as part of the outcome, we can cultivate profound changes.

CHAPTER 5

RESTORING ESTHETICS

She laughs at everything you say. Why?
Because she has fine teeth.

—*Benjamin Franklin*

MAUREEN CAME INTO MY OFFICE because her teeth were breaking and she was disappointed about their appearance. After walking her through the phases of Transformational Dentistry, we determined to rebuild all of her lower teeth as the first step in addressing her concerns. When she saw them in her mouth for the first time, she cried. Feeling slightly embarrassed by her demonstrative reaction, she asked, "Why am I crying?" I assured her it happens frequently in my office, and I explained how emotional it can be to feel whole again. Many patients don't give themselves permission to want that, but once they have it, they realize how significant of a burden they carried before the transformation.

Although every case has its unique elements and nuances, esthetics plays an integral role in almost every case I encounter. It's likely that I have not dealt with every person's unique combination of psychological, anatomical, and dental challenges but that's part of what I love about Transformational Dentistry—every case is a new puzzle. There are many factors that go with each patient, including psychological, financial, and time restrictions. These factors result in unique solutions for each individual, as we will see in the stories that follow.

In this chapter, we will look at the journeys of several of my patients who overcame multiple barriers in their paths to wholeness. They have helped show me the power of Transformational Dentistry, and they are the reasons I write this book. Their powerful evolutions began with their smiles, but extended into all areas of their lives. They inspire me daily, and I hope they can inspire you to take your first step on the path to wholeness.

STORY 1: SARAH

As I mentioned in Chapter 1, Sarah was one of the inspirations and catalysts for Transformational Dentistry. Her profound emotional transformation and the healing power of her new smile illustrate how emotions and dental care are interwoven. Sarah presented with a great concern about the appearance of her front teeth, which were worn out from stomach acid related to bulimia. In fact, her teeth were worn to the point that they were no longer in contact with her lower teeth. In cases of bulimia, the acid distorts the shape, color, length, and width of the teeth. This complicates getting the correct proportions of teeth so that the new teeth will look natural.

In Sarah's case, due to esthetic reasons, we had to perform a procedure called crown lengthening, which, given the length of her teeth was somewhat risky to do, because there was not a lot of root holding the teeth in the bone. If there's not enough tooth and you put a crown on it, it may fail. Her teeth became very loose after we did the crown lengthening, to the point that I was concerned that we might lose all of the affected teeth. In over a decade, hers is the only case where I've seen this happen. It's a singular instance that required careful management, so we decided to have her wear her prototype crowns for an extended period to establish the security of the teeth. Usually after crown lengthening, we wait a minimum of eight weeks, but in her case we waited closer to fourteen weeks.

Once the gums healed and the teeth were once again secure, we made impressions of her mouth and redesigned her teeth in the lab. Prototype crowns were placed on her teeth for several weeks, allowing us to evaluate her aesthetics, speech, and comfort in them. Once we were assured of the strength of her teeth, we put crowns on ten of her upper teeth to protect the teeth from stomach acid and to restore the esthetics. It has been several years now and Sarah's teeth are doing great. We don't have concerns about her losing teeth anymore. Her smile, like her body and mind, are healthy and strong.

Sarah's case highlights the importance of managing cases individually. Each situation must be considered in the context of the goals and the health of the individual. In her case, had we not been willing to push the boundaries a bit, she couldn't be where she is today. That's one of the real challenges that I see in the management of dental cases.

"Your face, smile, and eyes are the first things people see when they meet you. I saw my teeth slowly disintegrating over the years with clenching, grinding, and general erosion. Before my transformation, I didn't want to smile anymore. As my teeth were getting smaller and smaller, so was my self-esteem.

"Looking back, it was embarrassing admitting that I wanted/needed help—as Dr. Bishop wasn't the first specialist I approached. My smile has given me new confidence and I feel better about who I am. I'm me, but I think I look totally different when I smile, even now, years later."

—Sarah

Sarah Before Treatment

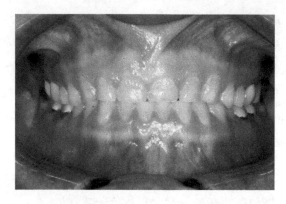

Sarah After Treatment

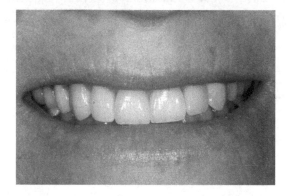

STORY 2: BONNIE

Bonnie's primary concern was related to the color and shape of the teeth. Bonnie had a job where she often appeared in TV advertisements, and she initially requested that we correct her smile by putting crowns on her upper front six teeth. With her permission, we thoroughly explored her concerns and desires about her smile before we committed to six crowns. As we did so, it became apparent that her trepidations were not solely related to the front six teeth, but rather to the entire smile. She came to understand that if we only addressed her front six teeth, it would draw more attention because of the stark contrast between her upper front teeth and the rest of her teeth. She also had discomfort related to her jaw joints, which was less burdensome to her than the esthetics, but I knew the pain would worsen over time.

Our initial step was to build up her lower teeth to a proper position to support her jaw joints. This relieved her jaw joint-related symptoms within a few weeks. Next, she had gum grafting performed to correct the "black triangle" spaces that had developed between her teeth. Once she had healed from this, we prepared all of her teeth for crowns at her new jaw relationship. She wore her prototype restorations for a period to evaluate the appearance, speech, and chewing functions. Once satisfied with these three elements, we completed the final crowns. The esthetic outcome was excellent. The biting relationship that she now has is more comfortable than she has enjoyed in decades.

Bonnie's case shows the real value in the Transformational Dentistry process. We accept a person's presenting concern, and in Bonnie's case, that was her smile; but as we dug a bit deeper, we discovered she had been enduring jaw issues for most of her life. It was evident that this was also a serious concern for her. The treatment plan that she initially requested ended up being totally inadequate for her because it didn't even address her facial and jaw comfort.

"All my life I was known for my big smile. Once I turned forty, the recession and upside down triangles in my smile worsened. After appearing in TV ads for my work, I would get emails asking me why I wasn't fixing the black marks on my teeth. They actually weren't black marks, they were spaces from over brushing. I began to not smile as much, and this did a number on my brain. I just accepted that this is the way it would be.

"I was having lunch one day with my friend, and thought something seemed different with her smile but could not figure it out. She mentioned Dr. Bishop to me, and I immediately booked an appointment. Since recreating my smile, my life is off the charts amazing! I truly did not even know this would impact my life so greatly. As soon as my treatment was done, Dr. Bishop gave me a mirror, and I broke down crying. These days, my cheeks hurt from smiling my face off 24/7."

—*Bonnie*

Bonnie Before Treatment

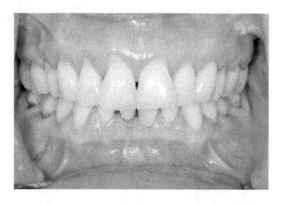

Bonnie After Treatment

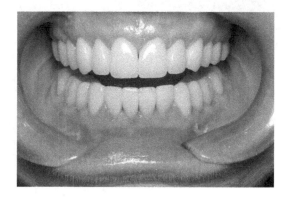

STORY 3: LONNIE

When Lonnie was a young man, he ground his teeth to deal with stress. He had the upper front teeth crowned to correct the damage. Over the ensuing decades, however, the porcelain of the upper crowns ground the lower front teeth flush with the gums. He also developed abscesses around his lower-right back teeth. We removed these abscessed teeth and prepared the bone to receive implants in six months. After six months, we also removed the lower front teeth and replaced all of the missing teeth with dental implants. After four months of healing, we redesigned his smile and then prepared his teeth for crowns. Prototype crowns were made for all of the teeth and the implants so that Lonnie could evaluate the function, esthetics, and speech with the proto-types. Once we were satisfied with these elements, we built the final crowns and placed them in his mouth. Lonnie was ecstatic about the outcome, espe-cially that his bite felt so good and that he could eat without discomfort.

> *"I'm sixty-three years old, and when I was in my thirties, I owned my own business and I ground my teeth off. My dentist at the time told me,*

'Here's a mouth guard, and you must wear it while you sleep because you're not going to stop grinding.' So, I've been wearing that mouth guard for forty years. About four years ago, I started losing my teeth on my lower right jaw. I had already lost one when I was a kid, and when you have a missing tooth, the other ones have no support. I went in and saw a dentist who told me it was time to have some major work done and referred me to Dr. Bishop. After extensive work, including a bone graft, extractions, and implants, Dr. Bishop put my new teeth in. They were beautiful. I really like them because I can chew on both sides now. My wife really likes them too. Recently, I saw a friend I hadn't seen for two years. We went out for lunch, and as I sat down and smiled, he said 'You got your teeth done.' I was surprised because he's not the guy you would think would notice. They're just absolutely beautiful teeth. I'm so glad I was patient. It was worth the wait."

—Lonnie

Lonnie Before Treatment

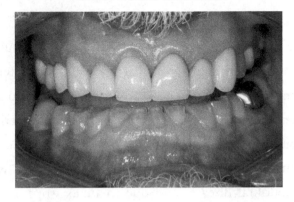

Lonnie After Treatment

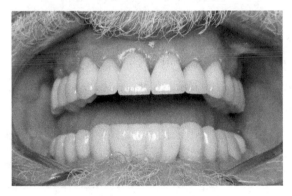

STORY 4: JULIA

When Julia presented, her primary concern was the esthetics of her upper front teeth, but in consultation with her, we decided that her failing lower teeth trumped her esthetic concerns. She had periodontal disease, which means she had a bacterial infection around her teeth that slowly erodes bone and gum tissue. There is a lot of systemic inflammation with periodontal disease, and due to Julia's work in the medical field, she was highly attuned to the cardiovascular impact of periodontal disease. So, although this was very much an esthetically driven case, she would soon be losing function of the teeth if not addressed. With periodontal disease, there's basically two ways of treating it: either clean the teeth regularly to remove the bacterial bioburden, or remove the tooth, which is more invasive, but sometimes necessary. Her lower teeth were at a point that they were compromised significantly enough that the decision was made to replace them.

Our first treatment was to remove the failing lower teeth and replace them with six implants and an immediate prototype restoration. Six months later when the tissues had healed around the implants, she received ceramic teeth to replace her lower teeth—

ideally for the rest of her life. She was excited about how good her new lower teeth looked and that she could eat more comfortably. A year or two later, she was ready to tackle her primary concern—the esthetics of her upper front teeth. An implant was positioned to replace the missing front tooth. We then redesigned her smile and placed prototype crowns on all of her front teeth so that she could experience and evaluate how the new teeth would affect her esthetics and speech. The prototype is critical to ensure we get the ultimate restoration right. She was very happy with them, so we reproduced the prototypes in ceramic. She now has a full and functional set of teeth and a beautiful smile that she is proud to share with all of the people around her.

"I have struggled with poor teeth my entire life. They were crooked, loose, discolored, and looked horrible. I really did not like to smile or talk. I knew my teeth [and the resulting periodontal disease] were making me very ill. One of my biggest motivating factors for having all the dental work done was that my daughter was getting married, and I wanted to have a beautiful smile for her special day. Despite the cost and some discomfort, seeing the transformation in my smile and feeling good

about myself was the best part of the process. I now have increased confidence. I am not afraid to smile or talk anymore. It was the best thing I have ever done for myself."

—*Julia*

Julia Before Treatment

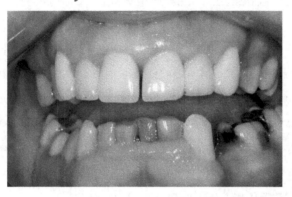

Julia After Treatment

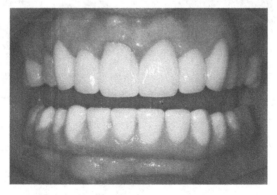

I hope you noticed a pattern as you read each of these stories. We call it Transformational Dentistry. We initially consulted with each individual and determined their needs and wants. After carefully evaluating the diagnostic records, we determined a course of treatment together. I hope you noticed that in each of these treatments there was a description of a prototype. The prototype is not a perfect representation of the designed smile, but it helps you to determine whether you will be happy with final result. The prototype can be modified; it can be remade. The prototype is a critical step in designing your new smile.

Often, people come to me for esthetic reasons, and they apologize or feel bad for being "vain." Having a smile you're proud of is not about vanity; it's about wholeness. If you feel this way, I give you permission to have a smile that you like to look at in the mirror. You deserve it. As I've learned from many of my patients, your smile is inextricably linked with your emotions—how you perceive the world and are perceived by the world. Don't get stuck in contrived barriers that are put on you by society, friends, family, or yourself. When you're seeking wholeness, it's a personal quest and a valid one. If part of your journey means having a beautiful smile, or a full set of teeth, then you should have it.

CHAPTER 6

CONQUER EDENTULISM

Peace begins with a smile.
—*Mother Teresa*

EDENTULISM IS THE state of missing some or all of your teeth. Edentulism has a huge impact on our nutrition, our psychological welfare, and our ability to show up with confidence in social environments. When someone loses a tooth, they often don't grasp the significance of the changes they might feel internally. Furthermore, one of the challenges with edentulism is that when you remove one tooth at a time, it is incremental; so the loss is not fully realized until there's significant loss of function. It can happen so slowly over a period of decades that one day you wake up, and you realize: I can't eat properly. I can't smile properly. I can't talk properly. It's a sneaky, crippling process.

People are far more responsive to the esthetic fallout from losing a tooth as compared to the functional fallout. Although, I would argue that the functional consequences are more significant long term than are the esthetic consequences in terms of overall health because when you cannot chew properly your nutrition and general health are compromised. People with edentulism will tend toward soft, squishy foods that are mostly processed and grain based, and not the most nourishing of foods. It's difficult to eat a steak without teeth. It's difficult to eat a raw carrot or a salad without teeth. I'm certainly not trying to downplay the esthetic consequences, which are significant to our psychological welfare, but for overall physical health, the functional loss is more significant. The goal of this chapter is to encourage people to optimize their state of health and wellness by overcoming the devastating effects of edentulism.

STORY 1: LORI

Lori presented to our clinic with an upper denture that she had been wearing for many years. She had three remaining lower teeth that were causing her pain. Although Lori is a small woman, she is tough. So tough, in fact, that she participated in competitions in which she strapped a harness to herself and towed a semi-trailer unit! Needless to say, she is a powerful woman. Yet, when it comes to dentistry, she was terrified. Her fear of dentistry was a huge component in her poor dentition. Luckily, her husband was supportive and present at all of the early treatment appointments, which helped her with the process. We removed the lower teeth to get her out of pain. We then designed her new smile and four implants were placed in the upper and lower jaws, for a total of eight. The same day, we attached her new prototype teeth to the implants. She wore these prototypes for six months while she healed. During this time, we made adjustments to get the bite comfortable and create improvements in the final set of teeth. It was a life-changing day for her. Six months later, we built the final set of teeth that would last for many years based on the changes that were created in the prototypes.

> *"For most of my life I endured ridicule and judgement by my peers and professionals because of my terrible teeth. By my fifties, my teeth had deteriorated until they weren't even functional anymore. I covered my smile a lot. My confidence deteriorated at the same rate as my teeth. I had to be particular about the food I ate because of*

poorly fitting dentures. Eating in public was very stressful for me because of my inability to properly chew some foods. I became extremely phobic of dentists and dental work. My phobia was so complete I could not walk into a dentist office because the smell was a trigger for me. I had to overcome this in order to set foot in Dr. Bishop's office for every step of this procedure. I spent a great deal of time with a therapist, who taught me breathing techniques. I was also at a point in my dental health where I had no other options but to do something to fix this.

"During one step of the process, Dr. Bishop asked me what I pictured my smile looking like when I was done. I had never been asked that before. I honestly couldn't tell him what I pictured because I had never thought of my smile ever looking any better. Now I can smile again with my whole face—a genuine happy smile that I am not ashamed nor embarrassed about.

"When you cannot smile, it changes people's perception of you. I no longer cover my face when I smile. I am not afraid to eat in public. I don't have steady tooth pain making some days unbearable. I can wear lipstick without

fear of it bringing attention to something I find ugly. Physically my whole world has improved tenfold.

"I catch myself looking at my reflection from time to time and tearing up. I went from spending my whole life not liking how I looked to looking in the mirror and feeling proud and grateful. Your smile, your teeth, are for more than just eating. Confidence and self-esteem affect all parts of your life, and if you can take that one step to fix what you don't like, it can change many aspects of your life. Do it."

—*Lori*

Lori Before Treatment

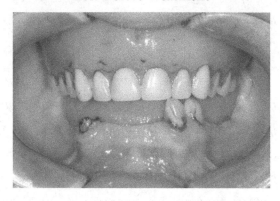

Lori After Treatment

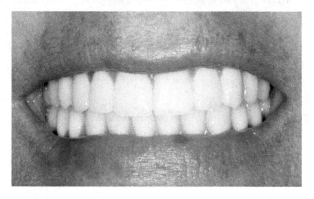

STORY 2: BARB

Barb presented with worn out teeth and two old partial dentures that were uncomfortable and esthetically distracting. She wanted a full set of teeth that would not come out of her mouth, so she could eat and smile with confidence. She had spent several decades building her business and raising her kids, and she was finally ready to obtain the smile she always wanted. We spent a few appointments designing her new teeth, after which four implants were placed in the upper and lower jaws to support the brand-new prototype teeth we built within twenty-four hours. After she had worn these temporary teeth for six months, we built her a new set with a few improvements that will last her for many, many years. Barb's case illustrates that there are ways of planning these transformations in stages, whether that is for reasons of comfort, time, finances, or pain.

> *"Before my dental transformation, I was inhibited, shy, and had lost a number of teeth. I was lacking in confidence and was embarrassed to smile. It was also difficult and painful for me to instruct classes and to talk publicly due to the partial plates. Having endured years of dental*

work for weak teeth, including painful partial plates held up with crowns that eventually broke, I was seeking a final solution to ongoing problems. I took the first step. I was committed to helping myself eat properly, feel confident, smile freely, be healthy, and enjoy a sense of freedom that comes with not being focused on the painful traumatic experiences of failing teeth.

"I can now do all of those things and just finished hosting a party for seventy people! Talking is no longer a problem, and being highly visible to others is a pleasure. The best part of the process was learning to smile again to show the beautiful transformation. I enjoyed seeing the change in myself. My new smile has affected my life in every way. I can chew and eat hard food again without pain. Salads are no longer a challenge nor are raw veggies. Smiling has meant I can go about my world and pass on the smile. It is said that when you smile the world smiles back, and it is true. You can elevate another's day just by the power of your smile. I can now talk freely in all situations and walk through my world with confidence.

"I still will look at the mirror and smile broadly at myself. It makes me feel happy, secure, and confident. I take pride in even brushing my teeth every day, thankful that I have these beautiful new teeth to care for. Do whatever it takes to get you to the solution. Life doesn't have to be focused on the past. Allow yourself to move forward in your own best interest. Dental work is so important and having the ability to eat without stress and with ease is so important to one's wellbeing. It's really the best thing I've ever undertaken on my own behalf."

—Barb

Barb Before Treatment

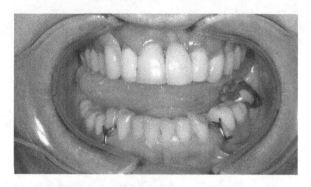

Barb After Treatment

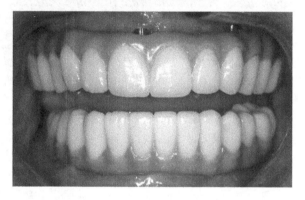

STORY 3: ANNE

Anne presented to our clinic because she was having severe jaw problems. She was wearing old dentures that did not properly support her jaw joints and face. Not everybody who loses teeth ends up with jaw issues that they recognize, but when you lose enough teeth, it always affects the jaws. She had a severely resorbed lower jaw that could not keep the lower denture stable. We placed two dental implants in the lower jaw to support her lower denture. New dentures, with porcelain teeth, were built with careful consideration for her jaw joint function using x-rays to measure the position of the jaws. Customarily, most dentures are built with acrylic denture teeth, but for someone such as Anne, we use porcelain teeth that will have greater long-term stability for her jaw joints, and thereby her jaw muscles, keeping her pain free for much longer. She has been functioning for years now without pain in her jaw joints and with much better function thanks to the implants.

"I was very self-conscious because my smile had worsened, but I didn't know what had happened. My lower jaw had changed my whole facial appearance. Before treatment, I was in a

lot of pain. It hurt to eat. Cold drinks made my chin feel numb, and I felt like I was drooling. I found it difficult to form my words correctly. I didn't enjoy socializing anymore and eating was often very painful.

"I think the hardest part about the process was the worry about how we could afford to do it. My nephew helped put the cost in the right perspective for me when he said, 'Isn't it odd how we spend thousands of dollars on new vehicles every few years but don't like to spend it on our jaws that are essential to us?'

"The best part was when a friend, who didn't know I was having this dental work done, saw me a week later and said 'Oh my goodness, you look different! You look so good. What did you do?' Another wonderful part of my dental work is that I no longer have any pain when I eat. I feel more relaxed around people and no longer cover my mouth when I smile."

—Anne

Anne Before Treatment

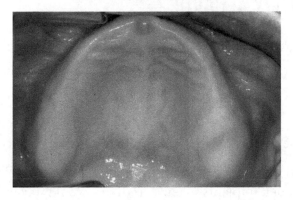

Anne After Treatment

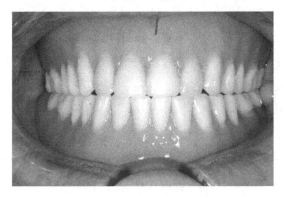

STORY 4: CAROL

Carol came to see me because she wanted to chew better. She was primarily concerned about function and wanted to replace her missing teeth with implants that would stay in her mouth. As we planned her case, we discovered that she had an abnormality in her lower jaw that would not allow us to safely place enough implants to build teeth that would stay in her mouth. She also had a front tooth that was severely out of position and had bothered her for many years. Until I asked her, "Do you have any concerns about your smile?" she didn't even think anything could be done with it. We redesigned her upper front tooth so that it would blend in. The lower front teeth were reshaped using crowns and veneers to fit with the newly designed upper front tooth. One implant was placed in the back of the lower jaw to support a partial denture that fit the new lower front teeth. With one implant and the new lower front teeth, the new partial denture fit almost like the teeth were designed to stay in her mouth.

Carol's case illustrates that one size doesn't fit all. Though the ideal solution would have been to use several dental implants to replace her missing teeth, she was not a candidate. We used a more traditional solution for her, one that fit her specific needs. Customization is required to meet each individual's needs. We used some modern techniques and some more traditional techniques; to solve everybody's problems, we need both. The process might be the same—figure out what they need, figure out what they want, plan tooth positioning, come up with a prototype, trial the prototype, and then deliver it—but the techniques can be vastly different, depending on each patient. Although she was primarily concerned about her function, she had this deep emotional desire related to her front tooth that had gone unaddressed for decades because she wasn't prepared and nobody asked. Carol came in just wanting enhanced function and ended up leaving able to chew better and having the smile that she's wanted forever but didn't think she could have. All it took was a little bit of creativity.

> *"Having spent quite a considerable amount of money on my mouth over several years, my smile was beautiful. Before meeting Dr. Bishop, I went for my usual dental check-up and was told that I needed surgery immediately or I could die. Apparently, there was a visible infection on the x-ray that came from my jaw. I was scheduled for surgery eight days later. When I*

awoke from the surgery, eight bottom teeth were missing—one of which was an anchor tooth, that supported a fixed bridge with three teeth. Also, on the bottom left, I was no longer able to support a bridge of four teeth. Dismayed by all these teeth missing in my mouth, I began my search for a new [dentist].

"It was awful walking around missing so many teeth. My self-confidence fell immediately! With many years of education and a wonderful career, I had come to the place of enjoying respect from others, including strangers. No doubt, in retrospect, a great smile and pleasant manner helped. But suddenly people didn't trust me or believe me. For example, store clerks wouldn't accept my return items. Not only were they looking at me skeptically, but they doubted me and came right out and said things like, 'Well this never happened before' or 'You must have broken it somehow.' Others just ignored me while I shopped.

"After the completion of my treatment, I can eat crunchy salads and other delicious foods. For most of my life, I took it as a given that I could not. My teeth now meet perfectly. I am

confident, friendly, and have high self-esteem again. Though I didn't do the actual dentistry work, I feel proud because my research and brains resulted in my choices! No one but you will determine how you will be able to live your best life."

—*Carol*

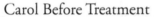

Carol Before Treatment

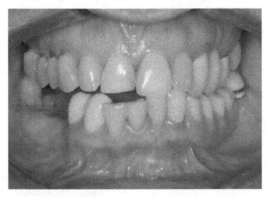

Carol After Treatment

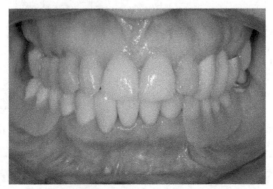

Emily came to my practice several years ago with decay and missing, crowded teeth. She wanted her teeth straightened to ultimately replace her missing teeth and get the pretty smile she always wanted. When she first came to me years ago, she had these lofty goals but poor self-care protocol. I sat her down and said, "You've got to change your habits and behaviors if you really want these things to be a priority. You've got to change." It took her a few years, but she showed up to see the hygienist consistently and set a new priority for herself. In doing this, she finally qualified herself to have orthodontic treatment, to get her teeth in the right place, so that she has a beautiful smile; we can now replace her missing teeth with implants. Years ago, she came with the inkling of a plan, but hadn't fully prioritized it. Over time, however, she qualified herself. What once was not possible for her is now possible because she chose a priority, she took action, and she is now going to reach her goals.

When it comes to dental care and function, you either prioritize it or you don't. I recently had a patient come in with compromised function. His girlfriend sat with him as we went over options. When he scoffed at the prices, she chimed in, "You've got $50,000 tied up in that truck of yours. You're in pain and you have no teeth! Why wouldn't you do this?" I understood her concern and frustration, but the reality is that this gentleman prioritizes the truck more than his teeth. This might change over time as he loses more function and his quality of life is further compromised, but I can't do anything to change his priorities. The patients in this chapter, however, decided that feeling whole and having a functional, esthetic dentition was a priority. If operating as a highly functional human being is important to you, then make allowances in your life so that you can achieve this. The path to wholeness begins with one small decision.

SMILE ON

YOUR SMILE IS INTEGRAL to the way you show up to the world. When you hide your smile, the world is missing one of the most important expressions of who you are. A smile expresses joy and warms other people. Every man, woman, and child deserves and requires a whole dentition for proper digestion, nutrition, expression, and confidence. These are basic requirements for a person to thrive in the community. In my practice, I have met countless patients who are seeking more than a solution to dental problems. They want their smile back; they want to eat with their friends at a restaurant; they want to have their picture taken without fear or anxiety about their looks.

One of the most common reactions my patients have after their Transformational Dentistry experience is, "I wish I'd done this sooner!" It is my hope that with some instruction and encouragement, more people will take advantage of the technologies and advancements available today. Now is the time.

In a world of international commerce and rampant advertising, there are many options available to solve problems. Dentistry is no different. One of the reasons I wrote this book is because I have met so many disappointed people who have spent thousands of dollars trying to solve dental problems, and they just end up disappointed with a failing solution. It's out of my frustration and sympathy for these people that I wrote this book in hopes of reaching them before they end up in a dire situation.

One of the challenges in our current healthcare paradigm is that we have become so proficient at managing and eliminating disease that we have lost sight of the true purpose of a healer, which is to restore the thriving vitality of the human body and soul. This book is part of a movement of healthcare practitioners attempting to unshackle and uplift the human spirit within our patients. My patients have inspired this movement within me, and I have witnessed their renewed vitality as a result of the restoration of their teeth and smiles. This is Transformational Dentistry.

Our modern society is busy and rushed. At Legato Dental Centre, we strive to take the time necessary to understand patients' wants and needs. Once we establish these, we are able to develop a winning plan for treatment and achieve results that consistently satisfy our patients.

Through the thousands of patients I have helped and the many other professionals I have taught using this revolutionary model of dentistry, it is my hope to build more dental facilities where human dignity is nurtured and developed through the maintenance, reconstruction, and replacement of teeth.

My invitation to you is to make the decision today to take a step toward a complete and esthetically satisfying set of teeth. For each of the patients who shared their stories in this book, it began with a decision that they were ready to solve their problem. Not all of them found the best solution quickly or easily; in fact, many of them had been through multiple providers just trying to find a reasonable option. My hope is that with this book in hand, people will be empowered and better equipped to make these decision for themselves in a more efficient and informed way.

I hope this book will motivate you onward in your journey to dental health and happiness. There is power in information, and I hope that in learning about the process of Transformational Dentistry, you will have the confidence to move forward and make the changes you want to make. Transformational Dentistry is not about the technical side of dentistry, but about the change that happens within the individual because of the metamorphosis that occurs within their mouth and mind through the process. Transformational Dentistry allows me to listen to my patients and address their specific needs. Every person is unique and, thus, every plan is customized for the individual. I am proud to support and empower patients and to encourage their involvement in the decision-making process. My hope is to connect with patients, educate them, inform them, and guide them through this transformational process that has dramatic effects on them physically, mentally, and emotionally. Never underestimate the power of a smile. Today is the day to take the first step toward transforming your smile, transforming your confidence, and transforming your life.

OUR SERVICES

At Legato Dental Centre, we provide a variety of services for our patients to get them the smile they deserve. We specialize in the following dental solutions:

- Tooth Replacement Options

- Esthetic Dentistry

- TMJ/TMD

- Sleep Apnea

https://www.legatocentre.com
(250) 860-5253

Printed in the USA
CPSIA information can be obtained
at www.ICGtesting.com
JSHW012040140824
68134JS00033B/3177

9 781599 329475